Coconut Oil Amazing Health, Skin and Cooking Benefits
Recipes Included

By
Gene Ashburner

ISBN-13:978-1502835789
ISBN-10:1502835789

Content

Coconut Oil - Amazing Health, Skin And Cooking Benefits

What To Look For When Buying Coconut Oil

Always buy Organic Virgin Coconut Oil.

Virgin coconut oil is unprocessed while refined coconut oil is processed. Unrefined coconut oil still retains the benefits of the fresh coconut.

Make sure the coconut oil is certified organic by USDA standards.

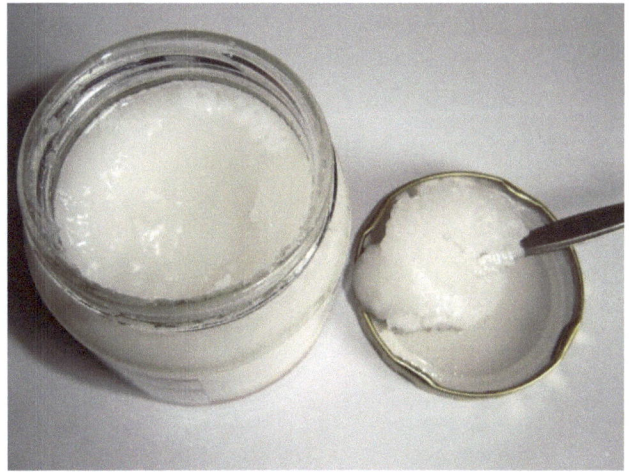

Make sure the coconut oil is made from fresh coconuts and not dried coconuts.

Make sure there are no chemical additives or preservatives added to the coconut oil.

Why Is Coconut Oil So Great

Coconut oil is more easily digested than other fats because it contains medium chain fatty acids. Medium-chain fatty acids are rapidly broken down and converted into energy putting less strain on the liver, pancreas and digestive system.

By activating the metabolism, coconut oil is outstanding for those with thyroid problems (over-active and under-active).

Coconut oil is antiviral, antimicrobial, anti-inflammatory, antifungal and anti-cancerous.

Coconut oil improves the immune system by destroying viruses such as HIV, herpes, influenza and pathogenic bacteria.

Coconut oil improves nutrient absorption.

Virgin coconut oil can be used both internally and externally.

Babies And Mums

Breastfeeding – Enrich The Milk Supply

Breastfeeding women should consume 3 ½ tablespoons of organic virgin coconut oil daily. The coconut oil will enrich the milk supply.

Cradle Cap - Remedy

Rub coconut oil onto a baby's scalp to cure cradle cap.

Diaper Rash - Remedy

Rub coconut oil onto a baby's bum to prevent diaper rash.

Nipple Cream - Remedy

Rub coconut oil onto the nipples. The coconut oil will nourish sore and cracked and dry nipples.

Baby Oil Recipe

Ingredients

1 oz coconut oil
2 drops pure lavender essential oil
1 drop chamomile essential oil

Method

Combine all the ingredients together.

Mix well.

Pour into a jar.

Coconut Oil Baby Wipes Recipe

Ingredients

1 roll strong paper towel
500 ml water
125 ml coconut oil
125 ml organic baby wash

Method

Cut the paper towel in half.

Take out the cardboard inner roll.

Combine the water, coconut oil and baby wash together.

Place one half of the roll into a container and pour over ½ of the solution.

Store the "wipes" in the container.

Cooking With Coconut Oil

Butter Substitute

Replace butter in recipes with coconut oil – the ratio remains the same.

Chocolate Substitute

37,5 ml cocoa powder mixed with 12,5 ml coconut oil = 1 oz chocolate.

Oil Substitute

Bake, cook or sauté food in coconut oil instead of using various other oils, butters, lards or fats.

Smoothies

Use coconut oil in smoothies as a nutritional supplement.

Chocolate Cashew Smoothie Recipe

Ingredients

37,5 ml virgin coconut oil
125 ml raw cashews

125 ml dates (stoned and chopped)
50 ml cocoa powder
375 ml coconut milk

Method

Combine the virgin coconut oil, cashews, dates, cocoa powder and coconut milk together in a blender.

Blend until smooth.

Serve immediately.

Chocolate Fruity Coconut Oil Snack Recipe

Ingredients

250 ml virgin coconut oil
250 ml cocoa powder
Dried cranberries
Dried blueberries
Raisins
Shredded coconut
Almonds (chopped)

Method

Combine the virgin coconut oil and cocoa powder together in a saucepan.

Heat until the coconut oil has melted and the mixture is smooth.

Mix well.

Add enough cranberries, blueberries, raisins, shredded coconut and almonds so that the mixture forms stiff dough.

Mix well.

Press the mixture into a greased square baking pan.

Refrigerate until the mixture has set.

Cut into squares.

Cherry Smoothie Recipe

Ingredients

250 ml vanilla yogurt
187 ml frozen sweet cherries
125 ml mandarin sections (drained)
37,5 ml virgin coconut oil
4 ice cubes

Method

Combine all ingredients together in a blender.

Blend until smooth.

Serve immediately.

Chocolate Fudge Recipe

Ingredients

50 g dark chocolate
75 g cream cheese
275 g icing sugar
35 ml virgin coconut oil
5 ml vanilla extract

Method

Melt the dark chocolate in the top of a double boiler, over hot water.

Beat the cream cheese and the icing sugar together.

Combine the melted chocolate and cream cheese mixture together.

Mix well.

Add the coconut oil and vanilla extract.

Mix well.

Pour the mixture into a greased pan.

Allow the fudge to cool and set.

Cut into squares.

Chocolate Sauce For Ice Cream Recipe

Ingredients

375 ml virgin coconut oil
95 ml cocoa powder
2 ml salt
7,5 ml coconut extract
95 ml pure honey
15 ml stevia

Method

Combine the coconut oil, cocoa powder, salt, coconut extract, honey and stevia together in the top of a double boiler, above boiling water.

Stir until the mixture has melted and is smooth.

Remove from the heat.

Serve over ice cream.

Coconut Banana Cake Recipe

Ingredients

2 ripe bananas (peeled and mashed)
62,5 ml desiccated coconut
125 ml virgin coconut oil
187 ml sugar
3 eggs
250 ml flour
5 ml salt
62,5 ml custard powder
250 ml virgin coconut oil
1000 ml icing sugar
25 ml sour cream
5 ml coconut extract

Method

Combine the bananas and desiccated coconut together.

Cream the coconut oil and sugar together until creamy.

Add the eggs to the sugar mixture one at a time.

Beat well after each egg has been added.

Sift the flour, salt and custard powder together.

Combine the flour mixture and the sugar mixture together.

Mix well.

Add the banana mixture.

Mix well.

Pour the batter into a greased cake pan.

Bake at 180 degrees C for 30 minutes.

Remove the cake from the oven and turn the cake out of the pan onto a wire cooling rack.

Allow the cake to cool.

Cream the coconut oil and icing sugar together until light and fluffy.

Add the sour cream and coconut extract.

Beat until the frosting mixture is light and fluffy.

Frost the cold cake with the coconut frosting.

Coconut Crunchie Cookie Recipe

Ingredients

250 g virgin coconut oil
12 ml golden syrup
5 ml bicarbonate of soda
100 g rolled oats
200 g sugar
160 g flour
50 g desiccated coconut

Method

Melt the coconut oil.

Add the syrup and bicarbonate of soda to the coconut oil.

Mix well.

Add all the dry ingredients to the coconut oil mixture.

Mix well.

Press the mixture into a square greased cake pan.

Bake for 45 minutes at 150 degrees C.

Remove from the oven.

Cut into bars while hot.

Coconut Ginger Smoothie Recipe

Ingredients

62,5 ml apple juice
37,5 ml virgin coconut oil
½ banana (peeled and sliced)
2 ml fresh ginger root (peeled and grated)
125 ml coconut milk

Method

Combine all the ingredients together in a blender.

Blend until smooth.

Serve immediately.

Peach Cranberry Smoothie Recipe

Ingredients

37,5 ml virgin coconut oil
250 ml peach yogurt
187 ml peach juice
125 ml frozen cranberries

375 ml peaches (peeled, stoned and chopped)

Method

Combine all the ingredients together in a blender.

Blend until smooth.

Serve immediately.

Peanut Butter Banana Smoothie Recipe

Ingredients

1 banana
30 ml peanut butter
125 ml coconut milk
25 ml virgin coconut oil

Method

Combine the banana, peanut butter, coconut milk and coconut oil together in a blender.

Blend until smooth.

Serve immediately.

Peanut Butter Coconut Fudge Recipe

Ingredients

1000 ml sugar
500 ml milk
3 ml salt
50 ml virgin coconut oil
10 ml vanilla extract

375 ml peanut butter

Method

Combine the sugar and milk together in a saucepan.

Bring to the boil.

Lower the heat.

Boil for 10 minutes.

Add the salt and coconut oil.

Continue boiling the mixture until the mixture forms a soft ball in cold water.

Remove from the heat.

Add the vanilla extract and the peanut butter.

Beat the mixture until it starts to set.

Pour the mixture quickly into a greased square baking pan.

Leave the fudge to set.

Cut into squares.

White Chocolate Cherry Fudge Recipe

Ingredients

50 g white chocolate
75 g cream cheese
275 g icing sugar
35 ml virgin coconut oil
5 ml cherry extract
125 ml candied cherries (chopped)

Method

Melt the chocolate in the top of a double boiler, over hot water.

Beat the cream cheese and the icing sugar together.

Combine the melted chocolate and cream cheese mixture together.

Mix well.

Add the coconut oil, cherry extract and candied cherries.

Mix well.

Pour the fudge mixture into a greased square pan.

Allow the fudge to cool and set.

Cut into squares.

Cosmetics Using Coconut Oil

Body Scrubs And Skin Exfoliators

If you want really soft skin, make your own body scrubs and skin exfoliators by combining coconut oil and sugar or sea salt together.

Deodorant

Rub coconut oil under the arm pits instead of using deodorant.

Eye Cream

Apply organic virgin coconut oil under the eyes to reduce eye puffiness, bags under the eyes and aging wrinkles.

Face And Body Moisturizer

Rub organic virgin coconut oil onto the face and body. Coconut oil makes a great face and body moisturizer as it will soften the skin. Coconut oil also contains a SPF to protect the skin from the sun.

Lip Balms And Lip Gloss

Rub coconut oil directly onto the lips. It will soften the skin and also the coconut oil contains a SPF to protect the lips from the sun.

Makeup Remover

Use coconut oil as a makeup remover.

Nail Strengthening Care

Combine a few drops of lavender essential oil with virgin coconut oil.

Rub the mixture into the nails to strengthen the nails.

Shaving Care

Rub coconut oil onto skin before shaving to prep the skin for shaving.

Rub coconut oil onto the skin after shaving. It helps for razor burn and does not clog the pores.

Soap

Make your own soap using coconut oil as the main fat in the soap.

Beeswax Coconut Body Butter Recipe

Ingredients

250 ml beeswax
150 ml baby oil
250 ml coconut oil
343 ml glycerine

Method

Combine the beeswax and coconut oil together in a double boiler.

Stir until the mixture has melted.

Add the baby oil and glycerine.

Heat until the mixture is smooth.

Remove from the heat.

Pour the body butter into a jar with a lid.

Beeswax Mango Body Butter Recipe

Ingredients

250 ml beeswax
250 ml coconut oil
250 ml apricot kernel oil
5 ml essential oil of choice
62,5 ml mango butter

Method

Melt all the ingredients together in a double boiler.

Mix well until the body butter is smooth.

Remove from the heat.

Pour the body butter into a jar with a lid.

Mint Body Butter Recipe

Ingredients

20 oz shea butter
6 oz sunflower oil
6 oz coconut oil
20 ml corn starch
2 oz peppermint oil

Method

Melt the shea butter in a double boiler.

When the shea butter has melted, add the sunflower oil, coconut oil, peppermint oil and corn starch.

Blend very well.

Remove the mixture from the heat.

Place the bowl containing the mixture into a bowl filled with ice water for a cold water bath.

This will help cool the body butter faster.

Whip the butter continually for several minutes with an electric beater.

Once the butter has solidified and forms peaks it is ready.

Pour the body butter into jars.

Coconut Sugar Scrub Recipe

Ingredients

500 ml sugar
250 ml coconut oil
25 ml shredded coconut
5 ml coconut fragrance oil

Method

Combine all the ingredients together.

Mix well.

Pour the sugar scrub into a jar.

Ginger Sugar Scrub Recipe

Ingredients

500 ml white sugar
125 ml coconut oil
125 ml almond oil
10 ml ground ginger
5 drops lemongrass essential oil

Method

Combine all the ingredients together.

Mix well.

Pour the sugar scrub into a jar.

Lavender Sugar Scrub Recipe

Ingredients

125 ml coconut oil
125 ml grape seed oil
250 ml white sugar
5 drops lavender essential oil

Method

Combine all the ingredients together.

Mix well.

Pour the sugar scrub into a jar.

Basic Lip Gloss Recipe

Ingredients

1 ½ ml paraffin wax (grated)
Ziploc bag
5 ml coconut oil
5 ml petroleum jelly
1 candy melt
0.63 ml oil-based candy flavouring
Grater

Method

Place the wax into the plastic bag.

Add the coconut oil, petroleum jelly and candy melt.

Add the candy flavouring.

Seal the plastic bag and place it into a bowl of hot tap water to melt the ingredients.

When all the ingredients are melted remove the bag from the water.

Mix the ingredients bag by shaking it gently.

Clip off a tiny corner of the bag and squeeze the lip gloss into a clean container.

Leave for 1 hour.

Use a cotton swab to apply the lip-gloss to your lips.

Lip Gloss Recipe

Ingredients

10 ml Aloe Vera gel
5 ml virgin coconut oil
10 ml petroleum jelly

Method

Combine all the ingredients together in a glass bowl.

Microwave the mixture for 1 to 2 minutes.

Mix well.

Pour the lip gloss into container.

Leave the lip gloss to cool.

Cherry Lip Gloss

Ingredients

25 ml beeswax (grated)
12,5 ml virgin coconut oil
2 ml vitamin E oil
2 ml cherry extract

Method

Combine the beeswax, coconut oil and vitamin E oil together in the top of a double boiler, above hot water.

Stir until the mixture has melted.

Add the cherry extract.

Mix well.

Pour the lip gloss into container.

Leave the lip gloss to cool.

Coconut Oil Face Wash Recipe

Ingredients

125 ml coconut oil
125 ml olive oil
125 ml almond oil
125 ml avocado oil
125 ml castor oil

Method

Combine the coconut oil, olive oil, almond oil, avocado oil and castor oil together.

Mix well.

Pour into a bottle and seal.

Digestion, Insulin Levels And Weight Loss

Cellulite

Coconut oil improves problematic cellulite. Rub the organic virgin coconut oil directly onto the skin as a moisturizer.

Cholesterol

Coconut oil improves the HDL to LDL ratio in people with high cholesterol. Drink organic virgin oil daily (see section - Recommended Daily Virgin Coconut Oil Dosage).

Constipation

Drink 1 to 3 tablespoons of coconut oil per day to relieve constipation and improve bowel function (see section - Recommended Daily Virgin Coconut Oil Dosage).

Diabetes

Coconut oil keeps blood sugar levels stable and helps with cravings. Drink organic virgin oil daily (see section - Recommended Daily Virgin Coconut Oil Dosage).

Dysentery

Dysentery is an intestinal inflammation that can lead to severe diarrhoea with mucus or blood in the faeces.

Coconut oil improves bowel function and inflammation.

Energy Boost

Coconut oil increases energy levels and endurance and is way healthier than eating chocolates or sugar laden snacks. Take a tablespoon of coconut oil when you feel your energy levels dropping.

Try doing this before a workout in the gym.

Gas Or Indigestion

Organic virgin coconut oil aids with digestion and gas or indigestion after eating. Take a tablespoon of virgin coconut oil before eating.

Insulin Levels

Coconut oil helps improve the insulin secretion and utilization of blood glucose.

Irritable Bowel Syndrome

Coconut oil aids with digestion and other digestion related problems such as irritable bowel syndrome.

Malnutrition

Coconut oil prevents malnutrition.

Metabolism

Coconut oil stimulates the metabolism and improves the thyroid function.

Thyroid Function & Hyperthyroidism

Coconut oil regulates an over-active or under-active thyroid. Drink 1 to 3 tablespoons of coconut oil per day (see section - Recommended Daily Virgin Coconut Oil Dosage).

Weight Loss

Coconut oil controls food cravings and increases the metabolic rate. Drink 1 to 3 tablespoons of coconut oil per day (see section - Recommended Daily Virgin Coconut Oil Dosage).

Hair

Chewing Gum In Hair - Remedy

Rub coconut oil over the chewing gum in the hair.

Leave the coconut oil in the hair for about 30 minutes.

Roll the chewing gum between the fingertips to remove the chewing gum.

Conditioner

Rub coconut oil into the hair and scalp.

Cover the hair with plastic and leave overnight for a deep conditioning hair treatment.

Dandruff

Rub coconut oil onto the scalp to prevent dandruff.

De-frizzer

Rub coconut oil into the hair instead of using a commercial de-frizzer.

Hair Loss

Coconut oil supports cell regeneration therefore if you apply coconut oil to the scalp it will prevent hair loss.

Head Lice

Coconut oil kills head lice – rub the coconut oil into the hair and scalp.

Leave the coconut oil in the hair for at least 60 minutes.

Rinse the hair with warm water.

Comb the hair with a nit comb.

Repeat 1 or 2 times more the following week to make sure the lice have been removed.

Dandruff Remedy Recipe

Ingredients

125 ml lemon juice
250 ml coconut oil

Method

Mix the lemon juice and coconut oil together.

Massage this oil onto your scalp (roots of your hair) before going to bed.

Hair Loss Remedy Recipe

Ingredients

125 ml coconut oil

125 ml castor oil
125 ml mustard oil

Method

Combine all the ingredients together.

Mix well.

Massage the mixture into your scalp (roots of your hair) before going to be each night.

Hot Coconut Oil Treatment Recipe

Ingredients

Coconut oil

Method

Heat the coconut oil in the top of a double boiler.

Remove the coconut oil from the heat.

Apply the warm coconut oil to the wet hair.

Cover the hair with a warm towel.

Leave for 30 minutes.

Wash with shampoo and rinse with warm water.

Health Care

Acid Reflux And Indigestion

Take a tablespoon of coconut oil after a meal to aid in digestion.

Adrenal Fatigue

Take the virgin coconut oil internally (see section - Recommended Daily Virgin Coconut Oil Dosage).

Allergies And Hay Fever

Rub coconut oil inside the nostrils for allergy and hay fever relief. The pollen will cling to the coconut oil.

Alzheimer's And Dementia

Take the virgin coconut oil internally (see section - Recommended Daily Virgin Coconut Oil Dosage) to prevent these diseases from occurring.

Autism

Coconut oil has proved to aid this problem. Take the virgin coconut oil internally (see section - Recommended Daily Virgin Coconut Oil Dosage).

Back Pain And Sore Muscles

Rub coconut oil onto the sore muscles and affected areas.

Boils, Cysts, Canker Sores, Warts, Athletes Foot And Toenail Fungus

Coconut oil will be affective in treating the following issues - boils, cysts, canker sores, warts, athlete's foot and toenail fungus.

Take the virgin coconut oil internally (see section - Recommended Daily Virgin Coconut Oil Dosage).

Rub the virgin coconut oil onto the affected areas.

Burns

Apply coconut oil directly onto a burn immediately after being burnt.

Thereafter frequently apply coconut oil while the burn is healing. The coconut oil will reduce the scarring and promote healing.

Cancer

Coconut oil has been shown to prevent colon and breast cancer in laboratory tests.

Crohns Disease

Coconut oil has proved to be effective in the treatment of Crohns disease. Coconut oil assists in the reduction of inflammation.

Take the virgin coconut oil internally (see section - Recommended Daily Virgin Coconut Oil Dosage).

Cuts And Scrapes

Apply coconut oil to cuts and scrapes – the coconut oil protects the wounds from dust, bacteria and viruses.

Coconut oil also speeds up the healing process.

Ear Infection

Drop a few drops of coconut oil inside the ear twice daily. The coconut oil fights the infection and also gives pain relief.

Epilepsy

Coconut oil is known to reduce epileptic seizures. Take coconut oil internally (see section - Recommended Daily Virgin Coconut Oil Dosage).

Genital Warts

Apply coconut oil externally on the warts.

If needed a coconut oil enema can be done twice a day, this depends on the location of the warts.

Heart Disease & Blood Circulation

Coconut oil protects the arteries from injury that causes atherosclerosis. Take coconut oil internally (see section - Recommended Daily Virgin Coconut Oil Dosage).

Coconut oil will improve blood circulation.

Hemorrhoids

Apply coconut oil externally or internally to the hemorrhoids.

Herpes

Coconut oil should be taken internally as well as rubbed on the herpes sores (see section - Recommended Daily Virgin Coconut Oil Dosage).

Hives

Apply the coconut oil directly on the affected areas. The coconut oil will reduce the itch and swelling.

Immune Related Diseases

Take the virgin coconut oil internally (see section - Recommended Daily Virgin Coconut Oil Dosage).

Coconut oil aids in the following health problems:

- HIV
- Immune System Builder

Kidney, Liver And Bladder

Coconut oil aids in the following health problems:

- Kidney Disease
- Kidney Stones
- Liver Disease
- Urinary Tract Infections
- See section - Recommended Daily Virgin Coconut Oil Dosage.

Lung And Respiratory Functions

A daily dose of coconut oil will address the following problems:

- Asthma in both adults and children
- Bronchial Infections
- Colds and Flu
- Lung Function and Lung Disease

- Coconut oil can also be used as a decongestant by rubbing it on the chest and under the nose.
- Oil pulling with coconut oil offers good health benefits.
- Nose bleeds – coconut oil can prevent nose bleeding.

See section - Recommended Daily Virgin Coconut Oil Dosage.

Mental Clarity

For mental clarity take the virgin coconut oil internally (see section - Recommended Daily Virgin Coconut Oil Dosage).

Migraines

With regular use of virgin coconut oil the migraines will crease. See section - Recommended Daily Virgin Coconut Oil Dosage.

Nausea

Rub coconut oil on the inside of the wrist and forearm, this will calm the nausea.

Osteoporosis

Coconut oil helps in the absorption of calcium and magnesium leading to better development of bones and therefore prevents and helps with Osteoporosis.

Drink coconut oil daily (see section - Recommended Daily Virgin Coconut Oil Dosage).

Pink Eye

Apply coconut oil in and around the eye.

Ringworms

Apply coconut oil directly onto the ringworms.

Sore Throat Remedy

Heat a teaspoon of virgin coconut oil.

Allow the coconut oil to slowly slide down and coat your throat.

Teeth And Gums

A daily dose of coconut oil will address the following problems:

- Periodontal disease and tooth decay
- Toothache
- For healthier teeth a daily dose of coconut oil will aid in the absorption of calcium and magnesium.
- Gum Disease and Gingivitis - rub coconut oil directly onto the gums. Make use of a coconut oil toothpaste.

Coconut Oil Aids Treatment & Prevention of the Following:

- Candida Albicans
- Chronic Fatigue
- Cystic Fibrosis
- Depression
- Rickets
- Scurvy
- Edema
- Fever Support
- Gallbladder disease and pain
- H. pylori
- Jaundice
- Mononucleosis
- Pancreatitis
- Parasites
- Thrush
- Ulcerative Colitis
- Stomach Ulcers

Take the virgin coconut oil internally (see section - Recommended Daily Virgin Coconut Oil Dosage).

Coconut Oil Toothpaste Recipe

Ingredients

100 ml virgin coconut oil
100 ml baking soda
15 to 25 drops peppermint oil (depending on your taste)
5 ml stevia

Method

Combine all the ingredients together.

Beat very well to get a light texture.

Store the toothpaste in a jar.

Dab the paste onto the toothbrush and brush as usual.

Swimmers Ear Recipe

Ingredients

2 ml ground turmeric
50 ml coconut oil

Method

Combine the turmeric and coconut oil together.

Mix well.

Drops a few drops of the mixture into the affected ear.

Repeat 2-3 times per day until the ear has healed.

Household Uses

Bronze

Rub coconut oil onto bronze household objects to clean the objects.

Furniture

Combine lemon juice and coconut oil together.

This makes a nourishing furniture polish for wood furniture.

Kitchen

Oil wooden chopping boards and bowls with coconut oil.

Season any new cookware with coconut oil.

Leather

Moisturize and clean leather products with coconut oil.

Cleaning Mixture Recipe

Ingredients

125 ml coconut oil
125 ml baking soda

Method

Combine the coconut oil and baking soda together.

Mix well.

Apply the mixture to the area that needs to be cleaned.

Leave for a few minutes.

Wash off with a sponge and warm water.

Massage And Stress Relief

Massage

Coconut oil works as a very effective massage oil.

Stress Relief

Coconut oil is extremely soothing thus helping to lower stress levels.

Men's Health

Prostate Enlargement

Take the virgin coconut oil internally (see section - Recommended Daily Virgin Coconut Oil Dosage).

Circumcision Healing

Coconut oil helps with the healing process use externally.

Pets And Coconut Oil

Add a daily teaspoon of coconut oil to your dog or cat's water bowl.

What Does Coconut Oil Do For Your Cat Or Dog?

- Improves the dog or cats general wellness giving a sleek and glossy coat
- Eliminates bad breath and odors
- Increases energy levels and normal thyroid function
- Helps to prevent or control diabetes in cats and dogs by regulating and balancing insulin levels
- Helps to reduce weight
- Helps with ligament problems
- Clears eczema, flea allergies, contact dermatitis, itchy skin, cuts, wounds and dry skin
- Improves digestion and nutrient absorption
- Helps in the elimination of hairballs and coughing
- Yeast and fungal infections - prevents and treats
- Treats allergic reactions
- Helps for Arthritis

- Digestive disorders - such as inflammatory bowel syndrome and colitis

Skin

Acne

Coconut oil improves and clears acne.

Take the coconut oil internally (see section - Recommended Daily Virgin Coconut Oil Dosage). Also rub coconut oil directly onto the face and affected areas.

Age Spots And Anti Aging

Coconut oil fades age spots – just apply the coconut oil directly to the age spots.

Coconut oil acts as a wrinkle reducer by strengthening the connective tissues in the skin.

Birth Marks

Coconut oil fades birth marks – just apply the coconut oil directly to the birth mark area.

Bruises

Coconut oil reduces swelling and redness on bruises – just apply coconut oil directly onto the bruise.

Dry And Flaky Skin

Apply coconut oil directly onto skin to soften and moisturize the skin.

Moles

Remove moles by first applying an apple cider vinegar compress then rub coconut oil onto the mole.

Do this for several weeks and the mole will disappear.

Oily Skin

Rub coconut oil on the oily T-zone area. This will reduce the oily appearance.

Skin Problems

Coconut oil relieves skin problems such as psoriasis, dermatitis and eczema.

Take the coconut oil internally (2 to 3 tablespoon per day). In addition to this you can also apply the coconut oil externally to the problem areas.

See section - Recommended Daily Virgin Coconut Oil Dosage.

Stretch Marks

Rub coconut oil onto stretch marks, it will nourish the damaged skin and help to improve the appearance of the skin.

Tattoos

Rub coconut oil onto tattoos to prevent the pigment from fading.

Rub coconut oil onto new tattoos to hasten the healing process and decrease the chance of infection in the tattoo area.

Pimple Cure Recipe

Ingredients

125 ml virgin coconut oil
125 ml thick curd
5 ml ground turmeric

Method

Combine the ingredients together to form a paste.

Apply onto the face to remove pimples.

Sun Tan Lotions And Insect Repellents

Bug Bites

Apply coconut oil directly onto a bug bite. It will stop the itching and burning sensation.

Insect Repellent

Combine coconut Oil and peppermint oil together.

Rub the mixture over exposed skin to ward off insects.

Sun Burn Remedy

Rub coconut oil onto the affected sun burnt area.

Coconut Oil Sun Tan Remedy Recipe

Ingredients

25 ml tea tree oil
250 ml coconut oil

Method

Combine the ingredients together.

Mix well.

Spread freely over the sunburned area.

It is soothing and pain-relieving and also reduces blistering and peeling.

Women's Health

Hot Flashes (Flushes)

Coconut oil is an effective remedy for hot flashes during menopause. Drink the coconut oil daily (see section - Recommended Daily Virgin Coconut Oil Dosage).

Lubricant

Coconut oil acts as a natural, safe personal lubricant. It is no compatible with latex.

Menstruation Relief

Take coconut oil internally to aid with menstrual pain, cramps and heavy blood flow. Drink the coconut oil daily (see section - Recommended Daily Virgin Coconut Oil Dosage).

Recommended Daily Virgin Coconut Oil Dosage

This chart is for persons over the age of 12.

Weight – Kilograms	Daily Dose of Coconut Oil
79+	4 tablespoons
68+	3 ½ tablespoons
57+	3 tablespoons
45+	2 ½ tablespoons
34+	2 tablespoon
23+	1 ½ tablespoons
11+	1 tablespoon

www.ingramcontent.com/pod-product-compliance
Lightning Source LLC
Chambersburg PA
CBHW040324010626
45792CB00024B/2116